BLOOD THINNING MEDICATION

201nm

Designed and written by:

Nester Kadzviti Murira PhD,M.Med.Ed.

This is a record of your health.

Carry this book wherever you go.

The information inside this book could save your life.

<u>Show this book to health personnel.</u>

Name:..

Address..

....

Tel..

Hospital/Dr..

Dr. 's Address..

....

Ambulance..

Allergies...

....

My Current Medication is:

1..

2..

3..

4..

5..

Why are you on blood thinning medication?

There are many reasons why the doctor may put you on blood thinning medication. The most common reasons could be that

- You have a weak heart
- You have had a heart attack before
- You have had deep vein thrombosis
- Your blood thickens because of some other reason

The blood thinners prevent heart attack and blood clots in the lungs and brain. Blood thinners prevent deep vein thrombosis.

How can one tell that their blood is thick and one needs urgent medical help?

- One can feel headaches
- Chest pain
- Intense body heat and sweating
- Cramps in the lower legs
- Body weakness

How does one suspect that one's blood is too thin?

- One feels heat especially in the center of the head
- One has pain in the thighs and one can actually see dark patches of bleeding under the skin of any part of the body.
- One has chest pain and feels heaviness in the chest.

Whether you feel as if your blood is too thick or thin, you must see health personnel immediately to have your blood checked for its thickness (INR) and have the blood thinning medication adjusted.

<u>Tests</u>

Blood tests to check thinness of blood must be done every month an the blood thinners regulated according to the blood thinness. The blood test enables health personnel to give you the medication according to the state of your blood.

<u>**Record the INR in this book**</u> every time it is tested.

Should you feel chest pain rush to the hospital and explain at the reception that you are on blood thinning medication. **Show this book to health personnel.**

Your chest will be examined for clots in the lungs and heart muscle.

- If you have a severe headache, a brain scan may be done to exclude clots in the brain. The tests are important in choosing the best treatment for you.

<u>Habits</u>

Smoking narrows and hardens blood vessels increasing the possibilities of blood clots. Smoking weakens the lung tissue and fills it with tarry substance from smoke that reduces absorption of oxygen. Your body becomes poorly supplied with oxygen. You need healthy lungs for good health.

Alcohol consumption

Alcohol interferes with medications and makes heart muscle weak.

Bathing

It may not be wise to soak yourself in a hot bath or sauna as this can cause blood clots especially in the legs.

A luke - warm shower is more comfortable and will not interfere with blood clotting.

Exercise

You can swim for short periods.

It is important to breathe fresh air and excise every day.

Take twenty minute to an hour walks every day to promote blood flow to your lower legs.

Weight: Keep average weight; weight gain strains your heart.

Pregnancy

Inform the doctor if you are planning a pregnancy or you think you are pregnant. Your medication may need to be adjusted.

Surgery

Before surgery, inform the surgeon that you are on blood thinners.

After surgery, move your legs as much as possible to promote good blood flow.

Your medication needs to be adjusted before surgery.

Dental appointment

Inform the dentist that you are on blood thinners when you make a dental appointment. Follow the advice provided by the dentist.

Diet

- Eat a well balanced diet.
- Eat plenty of fruit and vegetables as they contain vitamins and minerals that promote healthy blood. Fruit and vegetables contain roughage or fibre which promotes bowel movements and prevent straining your heart as you empty your bowels.
- Do not eat large meals at one sitting; your heart struggles to digest a large meal.
- Do not go to bed soon after a main meal. Eat your evening meal early and wait an hour or two before retiring to bed.

- Reduce fatty foods, salt in your diet, red meats, high starchy foods as these foods narrow blood vessels increasing the possibility of blood clots.

<u>Report</u> to hospital immediately if you have:

- Chest pain
- Bleeding under the skin and gums
- Excessive breathlessness
- Blackouts
- Swollen feet or face
- High temperatures
- Continuous bleeding after a bruise, dental check upor surgery.

<u>Rest</u>

- Give your body time to rest especially if you have a weak heart. Take a nap whenever you can.
- Always raise your feet on a stool or cushions to prevent swelling.
- Do not bend your legs or cross your legs for long periods
- Sitting on a hard chair may press hard on the blood vessels resulting in blood clots below the pressure.
- If you have a sedentary (sitting) job stand up every 1-2 hours and walk about to promote good blood floor around your body.

Travel

- See the doctor to have your medication doses adjusted in preparation for the journey.
- If driving, take a rest and walk about for a while before proceeding on the journey. Long drives cause poor circulation and clots in the lower legs.
- Drink a lot of fluids.
- Travelling by air causes thickening of blood. Walk around as much as possible while on flight. Drink plenty of fluids while on flight.

Medication:

Take your medication as advised.

- Do not skip your medications even when you feel well. If you forget to take your medications at the usual time, do not take a double dose.
- Do not take over the counter medications as some of them may interfere with how your medication works.

DATE	INR	MEDICATION ORDERED BY DOCTOR

DATE	INR	MEDICATION ORDERED BY DOCTOR

HAVE YOU TAKEN YOUR MEDICATION?

Tick in box after taking medication

Date/Day	Morning	Afternoon	Evening	
Monday				
Tuesday				
Wednesday				
Thursday				
Friday				
Saturday				
Sunday				

HAVE YOU TAKEN YOUR MEDICATION?

Tick in box after taking medication

Date/Day	Morning	Afternoon	Evening	
Monday				
Tuesday				
Wednesday				
Thursday				
Friday				
Saturday				
Sunday				

HAVE YOU TAKEN YOUR MEDICATION?

Tick in box after taking medication

Date/Day	Morning	Afternoon	Evening	
Monday				
Tuesday				
Wednesday				
Thursday				
Friday				
Saturday				
Sunday				

HAVE YOU TAKEN YOUR MEDICATION?

Tick in box after taking medication

Date/Day	Morning	Afternoon	Evening	
Monday				
Tuesday				
Wednesday				
Thursday				
Friday				
Saturday				
Sunday				

HAVE YOU TAKEN YOUR MEDICATION?

Tick in box after taking medication

Date/Day	Morning	Afternoon	Evening	
Monday				
Tuesday				
Wednesday				
Thursday				
Friday				
Saturday				
Sunday				

HAVE YOU TAKEN YOUR MEDICATION?

Tick in box after taking medication

Date/Day	Morning	Afternoon	Evening	
Monday				
Tuesday				
Wednesday				
Thursday				
Friday				
Saturday				
Sunday				

HAVE YOU TAKEN YOUR MEDICATION?

Tick in box after taking medication

Date/Day	Morning	Afternoon	Evening	
Monday				
Tuesday				
Wednesday				
Thursday				
Friday				
Saturday				
Sunday				

HAVE YOU TAKEN YOUR MEDICATION?

Tick in box after taking medication

Date/Day	Morning	Afternoon	Evening	
Monday				
Tuesday				
Wednesday				
Thursday				
Friday				
Saturday				
Sunday				

HAVE YOU TAKEN YOUR MEDICATION?

Tick in box after taking medication

Date/Day	Morning	Afternoon	Evening	
Monday				
Tuesday				
Wednesday				
Thursday				
Friday				
Saturday				
Sunday				

HAVE YOU TAKEN YOUR MEDICATION?

Tick in box after taking medication

Date/Day	Morning	Afternoon	Evening	
Monday				
Tuesday				
Wednesday				
Thursday				
Friday				
Saturday				
Sunday				

HAVE YOU TAKEN YOUR MEDICATION?

Tick in box after taking medication

Date/Day	Morning	Afternoon	Evening	
Monday				
Tuesday				
Wednesday				
Thursday				
Friday				
Saturday				
Sunday				

HAVE YOU TAKEN YOUR MEDICATION?

Tick in box after taking medication

Date/Day	Morning	Afternoon	Evening	
Monday				
Tuesday				
Wednesday				
Thursday				
Friday				
Saturday				
Sunday				